HASHIMOTO DIET RECIPES COOKBOOK

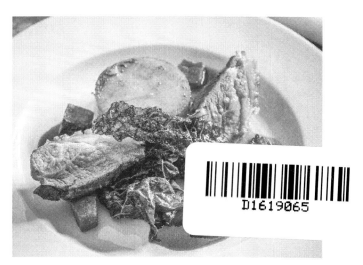

D1619065

Dr. Becca Smith

TABLE OF CONTENT

INTRODUCTION 7

CHAPTER ONE 9

Types, Causes and Symptoms of Hashimoto Disease 9

How to a Follow Hashimoto Diet and Benefits 12

CHAPTER TWO 17

14-Day Hashimoto Disease Diet Meal Plan 17

Day 1 17

Day 2 18

Day 3 18

Day 4 19

Day 5 19

Day 6 20

Day 7 20

Day 8 21

Day 9 21

Day 10 22

Day 11 22

Day 12 23

Day 13 23

Day 14 24

CHAPTER THREE 25

Hashimoto diet breakfast recipes 25

1. Berry Chia Seed Pudding 25

2. Spinach and Mushroom Omelette 26

3. Quinoa Breakfast Bowl 27

4. Sweet Potato and Kale Hash 28

5. Green Smoothie Bowl 29

Hashimoto Diet Lunch Recipes 30

1. Quinoa and Black Bean Salad 30

2. Grilled Chicken or Tofu Caesar Salad 31

3. Lentil and Vegetable Soup 33

4. Turkey or Tempeh Lettuce Wraps 34

5. Quinoa and Roasted Vegetable Bowl 36

CHAPTER FOUR 39

Hashimoto Diet Dinner Recipes 39

1. Baked Salmon with Lemon and Herbs 39

2. Turkey or Lentil Stuffed Bell Peppers 41

3. Chicken or Tofu Stir-Fry with Vegetables 43

4. Baked Chicken Thighs with Herbed Potatoes 44

5. Vegetable Curry with Chickpeas 45

Hashimoto Diet Dessert Recipes 48

1. Banana Oat Cookies 48

2. Coconut Chia Seed Pudding 49

3. Baked Apples with Cinnamon 50

4. Dark Chocolate Avocado Mousse 51

5. Mixed Berry Frozen Yogurt Bark 53

CHAPTER FIVE 55

Hashimoto Diet Snack Recipes 55

1. Almond Butter Energy Balls 55

2. Veggie Sticks with Hummus 56

3. Baked Sweet Potato Chips 58

4. Greek Yogurt Parfait 59

5. Roasted Chickpeas 60

Hashimoto Diet Smoothies and Juicing Recipes 62

1. Green Detox Smoothie 62

2. Berry Blast Smoothie 63

3. Pineapple Turmeric Anti-Inflammatory Juice 64

4. Tropical Mango Banana Smoothie 65

5. Beetroot Carrot Ginger Juice 66

CONCLUSION 69

INTRODUCTION

Alice had battled Hashimoto's disease for years, its symptoms often overwhelming her. Fatigue, weight gain, and a foggy mind seemed unshakeable companions. One day, weary of conventional treatments' limitations, she delved into the world of Hashimoto's diet.

With determination, she embraced a new lifestyle - gluten-free, dairy-free, and refined sugar-free. Her meals transformed into a vibrant array of fresh vegetables, lean proteins, and nourishing grains. Turmeric-laced dishes became her signature, its anti-inflammatory properties easing her symptoms.

Weeks turned into months, and the changes were subtle but profound. Alice's energy levels surged, her mind cleared, and the scale slowly tipped in her favor. Her perseverance wavered at times, but the encouragement from the supportive Hashimoto's community kept her going.

Unexpectedly, a year later, Alice found herself relishing a morning jog, something she hadn't imagined possible. Her journey with the Hashimoto diet had not only alleviated her symptoms but had also rekindled a zest for life she thought she'd lost. As she savored the simple joy of feeling healthy, she knew that her dedication to this diet was a life-changing decision worth every effort.

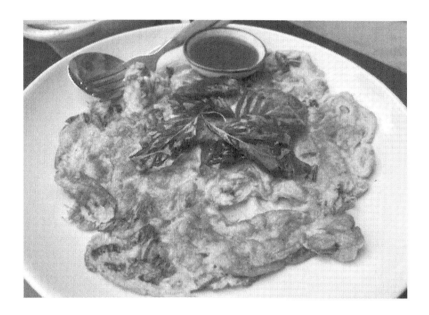

CHAPTER ONE

Types, Causes and Symptoms of Hashimoto Disease

Hashimoto's disease, also known as Hashimoto's thyroiditis, is an autoimmune condition that affects the thyroid gland. Named after the Japanese physician Dr. Hakaru Hashimoto, who first described it in 1912, this disorder occurs when the body's immune system mistakenly attacks the thyroid, leading to inflammation and eventual damage to the gland. This can result in an underactive thyroid, medically termed hypothyroidism.

Types of Hashimoto's Disease:

1. Classic Hashimoto's Thyroiditis: This is the most common form characterized by chronic inflammation of the thyroid gland.

Causes of Hashimoto's Disease:

1. Autoimmune Response: The exact cause is not fully understood, but it's believed to involve a combination of genetic predisposition and environmental triggers. The immune system mistakenly identifies the thyroid gland as a threat and produces antibodies that attack the gland.

Symptoms of Hashimoto's Disease:

1. Fatigue: Overwhelming and persistent tiredness, despite adequate rest.

2. Weight Gain: Unexplained weight gain or difficulty losing weight.

3. Depression and Mood Changes: Feelings of sadness, irritability, or anxiety.

4. Muscle Weakness: Generalized weakness, aching, or tenderness in muscles.

5. Joint Pain: Stiffness and pain in the joints.

6. Constipation: Difficulty passing stools or irregular bowel movements.

7. Dry Skin and Hair: Skin becomes dry and hair may thin or become brittle.

8. Sensitivity to Cold: Feeling excessively cold compared to others in the same environment.

9. Menstrual Irregularities: Changes in menstrual cycle or heavier periods.

10. Memory Problems and Brain Fog: Difficulty concentrating, memory lapses, or cognitive issues.

It's important to note that individuals may experience varying symptoms and their severity can differ widely. Diagnosis often involves a combination of physical examination, blood tests measuring thyroid hormone levels (TSH, T3, T4), and sometimes imaging studies like ultrasound of the thyroid.

Managing Hashimoto's disease typically involves hormone replacement therapy to address the hypothyroidism, and for some individuals, dietary changes (such as adopting a gluten-free diet), stress management, and regular monitoring by a healthcare professional to ensure optimal thyroid hormone levels.

Research continues to explore the complexities of Hashimoto's disease and potential treatments to improve the quality of life for those affected by this autoimmune condition.

How to a Follow Hashimoto Diet and Benefits

Hashimoto's disease, an autoimmune condition affecting the thyroid gland, can significantly impact one's quality of life. Fortunately, adopting a Hashimoto diet can alleviate symptoms and promote overall well-being. This comprehensive guide explores the principles, benefits, and steps to follow when embracing a Hashimoto diet.

Understanding the Hashimoto Diet:

A Hashimoto diet focuses on reducing inflammation, supporting thyroid function, and improving overall health. While individual responses to specific foods may vary, some general guidelines can benefit those with Hashimoto's disease:

1. Elimination of Trigger Foods: Many individuals with Hashimoto's find relief by eliminating gluten, dairy, and processed sugars from their diet. These foods can exacerbate inflammation and immune responses.

2. Focus on Nutrient-Dense Foods: Embrace whole, nutrient-rich foods such as vegetables (especially leafy greens), fruits, lean proteins, and healthy fats. These foods provide essential vitamins and minerals, supporting thyroid function and overall health.

3. Balanced Macronutrients: Strive for a balanced intake of carbohydrates, proteins, and fats. Healthy fats like omega-3 fatty acids (found in fatty fish, flaxseeds, and walnuts) and monounsaturated fats (avocados, olive oil) can reduce inflammation.

4. Mindful Eating and Stress Management: Incorporate stress-reducing techniques like meditation, yoga, or deep breathing exercises. Stress management can positively impact thyroid function.

Benefits of a Hashimoto Diet:

Adhering to a Hashimoto diet offers a range of benefits:

1. Reduced Inflammation: Eliminating inflammatory foods can decrease overall inflammation in the body, potentially reducing symptoms associated with Hashimoto's disease.

2. Improved Thyroid Function: Nutrient-dense foods provide essential nutrients that support thyroid health, aiding in the regulation of thyroid hormones.

3. Enhanced Energy Levels: A balanced diet can alleviate fatigue and boost energy, allowing individuals to engage in daily activities more effectively.

4. Weight Management: Proper nutrition and balanced eating can help regulate metabolism and support weight management, a common concern for those with Hashimoto's disease.

5. Enhanced Mental Clarity: A healthy diet rich in essential nutrients supports cognitive function, reducing brain fog and improving mental clarity.

Steps to Implement a Hashimoto Diet:

1. Consultation with a Healthcare Professional: Before making significant dietary changes, consult a healthcare professional or a registered dietitian familiar with Hashimoto's disease to create a personalized plan.

2. Food Journaling and Observing Reactions: Keep a food journal to track how different foods affect symptoms. Note any changes in energy levels, mood, or digestive issues after consuming specific foods.

3. Gradual Changes: Transitioning to a Hashimoto diet may require gradual changes. Start by eliminating one food group at a time to identify triggers and make the adjustment smoother.

4. Meal Planning and Preparation: Plan meals in advance to ensure they align with the Hashimoto diet guidelines. Incorporate a variety of nutrient-dense foods for balanced nutrition.

5. Regular Monitoring and Adjustments: Monitor symptoms regularly and be prepared to make adjustments to the diet as needed. What works for one person may not work for another.

Adopting a Hashimoto diet can be a transformative step towards managing symptoms and improving the quality of life for individuals with Hashimoto's disease.

By prioritizing nutrient-dense foods, reducing inflammation, and managing stress, one can positively impact thyroid health and overall well-being. It's essential to remember that dietary changes should be made in consultation with healthcare professionals for personalized guidance and optimal outcomes.

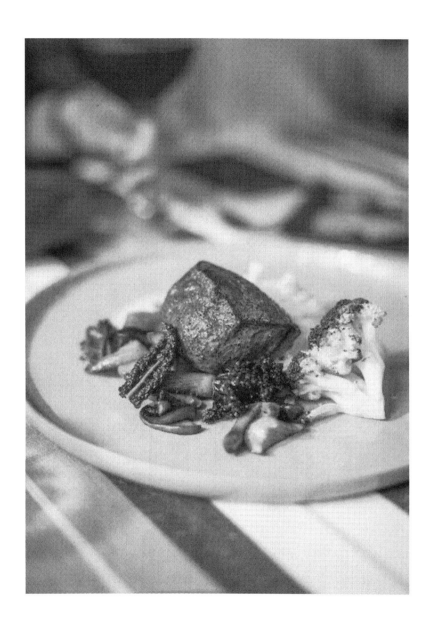

CHAPTER TWO

14-Day Hashimoto Disease Diet Meal Plan

Before starting any new diet, it's crucial to consult with a healthcare professional or a registered dietitian who can tailor the plan to individual needs. Here's a sample 14-day meal plan for someone with Hashimoto's disease, emphasizing nutrient-dense, anti-inflammatory foods while avoiding common triggers:

Day 1

- Breakfast: Gluten-free oats topped with berries, chia seeds, and a sprinkle of cinnamon.
- Lunch: Quinoa salad with mixed greens, grilled chicken, cherry tomatoes, cucumbers, and a lemon vinaigrette.
- Dinner: Baked salmon seasoned with herbs and served with roasted sweet potatoes and steamed broccoli.

Day 2

- Breakfast: Greek yogurt (dairy-free if preferred) with sliced bananas, almonds, and a drizzle of honey.
- Lunch: Lentil soup with carrots, celery, and spinach. Served with a side of gluten-free crackers or a small quinoa salad.
- Dinner: Turkey chili made with lean ground turkey, kidney beans, tomatoes, and spices. Serve with a side of sautéed greens.

Day 3

- Breakfast: Smoothie with spinach, frozen berries, almond milk, hemp seeds, and a scoop of protein powder (gluten-free and dairy-free).
- Lunch: Brown rice stir-fry with tofu or chicken, mixed vegetables, and a homemade teriyaki sauce (without gluten).
- Dinner: Grilled chicken breast with a side of roasted root vegetables (carrots, beets, parsnips) and a mixed green salad.

Day 4

- Breakfast: Scrambled eggs with sautéed spinach, tomatoes, and avocado on gluten-free toast or a rice cake.
- Lunch: Quinoa and black bean salad with diced bell peppers, corn, cilantro, and a lime-cumin dressing.
- Dinner: Baked cod fillet with a side of quinoa pilaf and steamed asparagus.

Day 5

- Breakfast: Chia seed pudding made with almond milk, topped with fresh fruit and sliced almonds.
- Lunch: Mixed greens salad with grilled shrimp, avocado, cherry tomatoes, and a balsamic vinaigrette.
- Dinner: Beef or tempeh (for vegetarians/vegans) lettuce wraps with a variety of vegetables and a ginger-soy sauce.

Day 6

- Breakfast: Smoothie bowl topped with granola, sliced fruits, coconut flakes, and pumpkin seeds.
- Lunch: Turkey or tofu (for vegetarians/vegans) lettuce cups with diced veggies and a tahini dressing.
- Dinner: Baked chicken thighs with roasted Brussels sprouts and a quinoa-stuffed bell pepper.

Day 7

- Breakfast: Almond flour pancakes topped with berries and a drizzle of pure maple syrup.
- Lunch: Lentil and vegetable soup with a side of gluten-free bread or crackers.
- Dinner: Grilled steak or portobello mushrooms (for vegetarians/vegans) with roasted sweet potatoes and a kale salad.

Day 8

- Breakfast: Smoothie with spinach, frozen mango, almond milk, flaxseeds, and a scoop of protein powder.
- Lunch: Quinoa and roasted vegetable salad with chickpeas, red bell peppers, zucchini, and a lemon-tahini dressing.
- Dinner: Baked cod or tofu (for vegetarians/vegans) with a side of wild rice pilaf and steamed green beans.

Day 9

- Breakfast: Buckwheat pancakes topped with sliced bananas, walnuts, and a drizzle of honey or pure maple syrup.
- Lunch: Chicken or tempeh (for vegetarians/vegans) Caesar salad with romaine lettuce, homemade dressing, and gluten-free croutons.
- Dinner: Spaghetti squash with marinara sauce and turkey meatballs or lentil meatballs for a vegetarian option. Serve with a side salad.

Day 10

- Breakfast: Avocado toast on gluten-free bread or rice cakes with cherry tomatoes and a sprinkle of hemp seeds.
- Lunch: Grilled shrimp or marinated tofu (for vegetarians/vegans) skewers with bell peppers, onions, and a quinoa tabbouleh.
- Dinner: Stir-fried beef or tempeh (for vegetarians/vegans) with broccoli, bell peppers, and a homemade ginger-garlic sauce, served over brown rice.

Day 11

- Breakfast: Chia seed pudding made with coconut milk, topped with mixed berries and shredded coconut.
- Lunch: Greek salad with cucumber, olives, cherry tomatoes, feta cheese or a dairy-free alternative, and grilled chicken or tofu.
- Dinner: Baked halibut or portobello mushrooms (for vegetarians/vegans) with quinoa pilaf and roasted cauliflower.

Day 12

- Breakfast: Breakfast burrito with scrambled eggs or tofu (for vegetarians/vegans), black beans, avocado, and salsa wrapped in a gluten-free tortilla.
- Lunch: Turkey or tempeh (for vegetarians/vegans) lettuce wraps with a variety of crunchy vegetables and a sesame-ginger dressing.
- Dinner: Lemon-herb roasted chicken thighs with sweet potato mash and steamed broccoli.

Day 13

- Breakfast: Green smoothie with kale, pineapple, banana, coconut water, and a scoop of plant-based protein powder.
- Lunch: Quinoa-stuffed bell peppers with black beans, corn, and spices, served with a side of mixed greens.
- Dinner: Grilled salmon or marinated tempeh (for vegetarians/vegans) with roasted root vegetables and a mixed green salad.

Day 14

- Breakfast: Overnight oats with almond milk, grated apple, cinnamon, and a handful of nuts and seeds.
- Lunch: Lentil and vegetable curry served over brown rice or quinoa.
- Dinner: Turkey or tofu (for vegetarians/vegans) taco bowls with lettuce, black beans, tomatoes, avocado, and salsa.

This two-week meal plan provides a variety of nutrient-dense, anti-inflammatory meals suitable for individuals with Hashimoto's disease. Adjust portions and ingredients based on personal preferences and dietary needs while ensuring a balanced intake of nutrients.

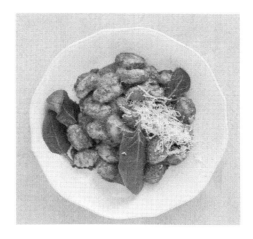

CHAPTER THREE

Hashimoto diet breakfast recipes

Starting your day with a nutritious breakfast is crucial, especially for individuals managing Hashimoto's disease. These five breakfast recipes are designed to provide a balance of nutrients, supporting thyroid health while being delicious and easy to prepare.

1. Berry Chia Seed Pudding

Ingredients:

- 1/4 cup chia seeds
- 1 cup unsweetened almond milk (or any preferred milk)
- 1/2 teaspoon vanilla extract
- 1 tablespoon maple syrup (optional)
- Mixed berries for topping

Instructions:

1. In a bowl or jar, mix chia seeds, almond milk, vanilla extract, and maple syrup (if using). Stir well.

2. Cover and refrigerate overnight or for at least 4 hours, allowing the chia seeds to expand and create a pudding-like consistency.

3. Before serving, stir the mixture again and top with fresh mixed berries.

Cooking Time: 5 minutes prep + refrigeration time

2. Spinach and Mushroom Omelette

Ingredients:

- 2 large eggs
- 1 cup fresh spinach, chopped
- 1/2 cup mushrooms, sliced
- 1 tablespoon olive oil or coconut oil
- Salt and pepper to taste

Instructions:

1. Heat oil in a non-stick skillet over medium heat.

2. Sauté mushrooms until they soften, then add chopped spinach and cook until wilted. Season with salt and pepper.

3. In a bowl, beat eggs and pour them into the skillet over the cooked vegetables.

4. Cook the omelette until the eggs are set, then fold it in half and slide it onto a plate.

Cooking Time: 10 minutes

3. Quinoa Breakfast Bowl

Ingredients:

- 1/2 cup cooked quinoa
- 1/4 cup sliced almonds
- 1/2 cup mixed berries (blueberries, raspberries)
- 1 tablespoon honey or maple syrup (optional)
- Greek yogurt (dairy-free if preferred)

Instructions:

1. In a bowl, layer cooked quinoa, sliced almonds, and mixed berries.

2. Drizzle with honey or maple syrup if desired and serve with a dollop of Greek yogurt on top.

Cooking Time: 5 minutes (if quinoa is pre-cooked)

4. Sweet Potato and Kale Hash

Ingredients:

- 1 medium sweet potato, diced
- 1 cup kale, chopped
- 1/2 onion, diced
- 2 tablespoons olive oil
- Salt, pepper, and paprika to taste

Instructions:

1. Heat olive oil in a skillet over medium heat. Add diced sweet potatoes and onions. Cook until sweet potatoes are tender and slightly browned.

2. Add chopped kale to the skillet and cook until wilted. Season with salt, pepper, and paprika.

3. Serve the sweet potato and kale hash as a nutritious breakfast side dish.

Cooking Time: 15-20 minutes

5. Green Smoothie Bowl

Ingredients:

- 1 ripe banana, frozen
- 1 cup spinach or kale
- 1/2 avocado
- 1/2 cup unsweetened almond milk (or any preferred milk)
- Toppings: sliced fruits, granola, chia seeds, shredded coconut

Instructions:

1. Blend banana, spinach or kale, avocado, and almond milk until smooth.

2. Pour the smoothie into a bowl and top it with your favorite fruits, granola, chia seeds, and shredded coconut.

Cooking Time: 5 minutes

These breakfast recipes offer variety and nutrition, aligning with a Hashimoto's diet. They are easy to customize and are packed with essential nutrients to kickstart your day on a healthy note.

Hashimoto Diet Lunch Recipes

Here are five lunch recipes tailored to the Hashimoto's diet, aiming to provide balanced nutrition and delicious options that support thyroid health.

1. Quinoa and Black Bean Salad

This vibrant and protein-packed salad is a perfect addition to your Hashimoto's diet lunch. It's filled with nutrient-rich ingredients that support thyroid function and overall well-being.

Ingredients:

- 1 cup cooked quinoa
- 1 can black beans, rinsed and drained
- 1 red bell pepper, diced
- 1/2 red onion, finely chopped
- 1/4 cup chopped fresh cilantro
- Juice of 1 lime
- 2 tablespoons olive oil
- Salt and pepper to taste

Instructions:

1. In a large bowl, combine cooked quinoa, black beans, diced bell pepper, chopped onion, and cilantro.

2. In a separate small bowl, whisk together lime juice, olive oil, salt, and pepper to create the dressing.

3. Pour the dressing over the salad and toss gently to combine.

4. Serve chilled or at room temperature.

Cooking Time: 15 minutes

2. Grilled Chicken or Tofu Caesar Salad

This Caesar salad is a wholesome and flavorful lunch option. The homemade dressing and fresh ingredients make it a perfect choice for a satisfying and thyroid-friendly meal.

Ingredients:

- Grilled chicken breast or tofu slices (for vegetarians/vegans)
- Romaine lettuce, chopped

- Gluten-free croutons
- Dairy-free Caesar dressing (made with olive oil, lemon juice, garlic, Dijon mustard, and anchovy paste or alternative)

Instructions:

1. Prepare the grilled chicken or tofu according to your preference.

2. In a large bowl, toss chopped romaine lettuce with gluten-free croutons.

3. Add grilled chicken or tofu on top of the salad.

4. Drizzle the Caesar dressing over the salad and toss gently to coat.

Cooking Time: Depends on grilling method (approximately 15-20 minutes)

3. Lentil and Vegetable Soup

This hearty soup is packed with fiber and essential nutrients, making it an ideal lunch for those with Hashimoto's disease. It's nourishing, comforting, and supports a balanced diet.

Ingredients:

- 1 cup green or brown lentils, rinsed
- 4 cups vegetable or chicken broth
- 1 onion, diced
- 2 carrots, chopped
- 2 celery stalks, chopped
- 2 cloves garlic, minced
- 1 teaspoon dried thyme
- Salt and pepper to taste
- Fresh parsley for garnish

Instructions:

1. In a large pot, sauté diced onion, carrots, celery, and garlic until softened.

2. Add lentils, vegetable or chicken broth, dried thyme, salt, and pepper. Bring to a boil, then reduce heat and simmer for 25-30 minutes until lentils are tender.

3. Serve hot, garnished with fresh parsley.

Cooking Time: 35-40 minutes

4. Turkey or Tempeh Lettuce Wraps

These lettuce wraps are a light yet satisfying lunch option. Packed with protein and fresh flavors, they're perfect for a Hashimoto's diet.

Ingredients:

- Ground turkey or crumbled tempeh (for vegetarians/vegans)
- Lettuce leaves (butterhead or iceberg)
- 1 tablespoon olive oil
- Minced garlic

- Diced bell peppers, water chestnuts, and mushrooms
- Low-sodium soy sauce or tamari
- Fresh cilantro for garnish

Instructions:

1. In a skillet, heat olive oil and sauté minced garlic until fragrant.

2. Add ground turkey or crumbled tempeh and cook until browned.

3. Stir in diced bell peppers, water chestnuts, and mushrooms. Cook until vegetables are tender.

4. Season with low-sodium soy sauce or tamari.

5. Spoon the mixture into lettuce leaves, garnish with fresh cilantro, and serve.

Cooking Time: Approximately 15 minutes

5. Quinoa and Roasted Vegetable Bowl

This versatile and colorful bowl combines roasted vegetables with quinoa for a satisfying and nutrient-rich lunch, perfect for supporting a Hashimoto's diet.

Ingredients:

- Roasted vegetables (bell peppers, zucchini, eggplant, cherry tomatoes)
- Cooked quinoa
- Olive oil
- Herbs and spices (such as thyme, rosemary, garlic powder)
- Salt and pepper to taste
- Optional: a drizzle of balsamic glaze

Instructions:

1. Preheat the oven to 400°F (200°C).

2. Toss chopped vegetables with olive oil, herbs, spices, salt, and pepper.

3. Roast the vegetables in the oven for 20-25 minutes until tender and slightly caramelized.

4. Assemble the bowl with cooked quinoa as the base and top it with roasted vegetables.

5. Drizzle with a little balsamic glaze for extra flavor if desired.

Cooking Time: Approximately 30 minutes (including vegetable roasting time)

These lunch recipes offer a range of flavors and nutrients while aligning with the principles of a Hashimoto's diet. Adjust ingredients according to preferences and dietary needs for a nourishing and enjoyable lunch experience.

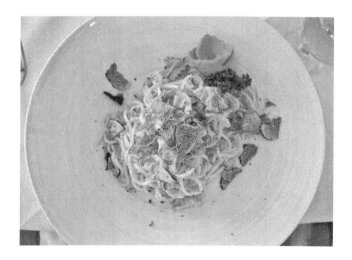

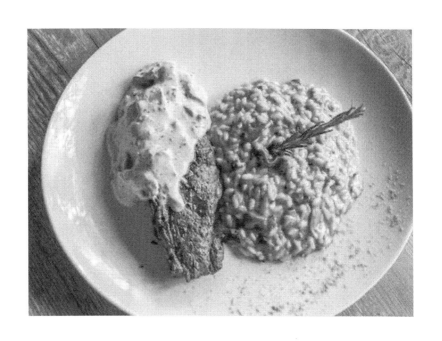

CHAPTER FOUR

Hashimoto Diet Dinner Recipes

Absolutely! Here are five dinner recipes suitable for a Hashimoto's diet. Each dish is designed to be flavorful, nutritious, and supportive of thyroid health.

1. Baked Salmon with Lemon and Herbs

This baked salmon dish is rich in omega-3 fatty acids and protein, supporting thyroid function. The addition of lemon and herbs adds a burst of flavor to this simple and nutritious dinner option.

Ingredients:

- 4 salmon fillets
- 2 tablespoons olive oil
- 2 tablespoons fresh lemon juice
- 2 cloves garlic, minced
- 1 teaspoon dried dill
- Salt and pepper to taste
- Lemon slices for garnish
- Fresh parsley for garnish

Instructions:

1. Preheat the oven to 375°F (190°C) and line a baking dish with parchment paper.

2. Place the salmon fillets in the baking dish.

3. In a small bowl, mix olive oil, lemon juice, minced garlic, dried dill, salt, and pepper.

4. Pour the mixture over the salmon fillets, ensuring they are evenly coated.

5. Bake for 12-15 minutes or until the salmon is cooked through and flakes easily with a fork.

6. Garnish with lemon slices and fresh parsley before serving.

Cooking Time: 15 minutes

2. Turkey or Lentil Stuffed Bell Peppers

These stuffed bell peppers are a hearty and versatile dinner option, offering a balanced mix of protein and vegetables. They can be made with either ground turkey or lentils for a vegetarian/vegan alternative.

Ingredients:

- Bell peppers (any color), halved and seeds removed
- 1 cup cooked quinoa or rice
- Ground turkey or cooked lentils
- Onion, diced
- Garlic, minced
- Diced tomatoes
- Italian seasoning
- Salt and pepper to taste
- Shredded cheese or dairy-free cheese (optional)

Instructions:

1. Preheat the oven to 375°F (190°C) and prepare the bell peppers in a baking dish.

2. In a skillet, sauté onion and garlic until softened. Add ground turkey or cooked lentils and cook until browned or heated through.

3. Stir in diced tomatoes, cooked quinoa or rice, Italian seasoning, salt, and pepper. Mix well.

4. Spoon the filling into the bell pepper halves.

5. If using cheese, sprinkle it on top of the stuffed peppers.

6. Bake for 25-30 minutes or until the peppers are tender.

Cooking Time: Approximately 35-40 minutes (including baking time)

3. Chicken or Tofu Stir-Fry with Vegetables

This stir-fry is a quick and versatile dinner choice that can be made with chicken or tofu, providing protein and a variety of vegetables for essential nutrients.

Ingredients:

- Chicken breast strips or cubed tofu
- Mixed vegetables (bell peppers, broccoli, carrots, snow peas)
- Garlic, minced
- Ginger, grated
- Low-sodium soy sauce or tamari
- Sesame oil
- Brown rice or quinoa (optional, for serving)

Instructions:

1. In a wok or large skillet, heat sesame oil over medium-high heat.

2. Add minced garlic and grated ginger, sautéing until fragrant.

3. Add chicken strips or tofu cubes, cooking until they are browned or heated through.

4. Toss in the mixed vegetables and stir-fry until they are tender yet crisp.

5. Drizzle with low-sodium soy sauce or tamari and toss to coat evenly.

6. Serve over brown rice or quinoa if desired.

Cooking Time: Approximately 15-20 minutes

4. Baked Chicken Thighs with Herbed Potatoes

This dinner recipe pairs tender baked chicken thighs with flavorful herbed potatoes, offering a satisfying and well-rounded meal for individuals on a Hashimoto's diet.

Ingredients:

- Chicken thighs, bone-in and skin-on
- Baby potatoes, halved
- Olive oil
- Fresh rosemary, thyme, and parsley (or dried herbs)

- Garlic powder
- Salt and pepper to taste

Instructions:

1. Preheat the oven to 400°F (200°C).

2. Place chicken thighs on a baking sheet lined with parchment paper.

3. In a bowl, toss halved baby potatoes with olive oil, herbs, garlic powder, salt, and pepper.

4. Arrange the seasoned potatoes around the chicken thighs on the baking sheet.

5. Bake for 35-40 minutes or until the chicken is cooked through and the potatoes are golden brown and tender.

Cooking Time: 40 minutes

5. Vegetable Curry with Chickpeas

This vegetable curry is a comforting and flavorful dinner option packed with colorful vegetables, chickpeas for protein, and aromatic spices. It's a great addition to a Hashimoto's diet due to its nutrient density.

Ingredients:

- Assorted vegetables (such as bell peppers, carrots, cauliflower, peas)
- Chickpeas (canned or cooked)
- Onion, diced
- Garlic, minced
- Ginger, grated
- Curry powder or paste
- Coconut milk
- Vegetable broth
- Fresh cilantro for garnish
- Brown rice or quinoa (optional, for serving)

Instructions:

1. In a pot or large skillet, sauté diced onion, minced garlic, and grated ginger until softened.

2. Add assorted vegetables and chickpeas, stirring to combine.

3. Stir in curry powder or paste and cook for a minute to release flavors.

4. Pour in coconut milk and vegetable broth, bringing the mixture to a simmer.

5. Cover and let it simmer for 15-20 minutes until the vegetables are tender.

6. Serve the vegetable curry over brown rice or quinoa and garnish with fresh cilantro.

Cooking Time: Approximately 30-35 minutes

These dinner recipes offer a variety of flavors and nutrients while aligning with the principles of a Hashimoto's diet. Adjust ingredients according to preferences and dietary needs for a nourishing and enjoyable dinner experience.

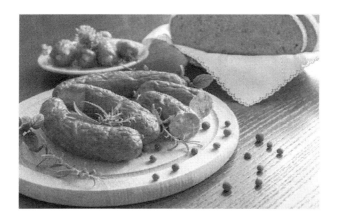

Hashimoto Diet Dessert Recipes

1. Banana Oat Cookies

These banana oat cookies are a delightful treat that's easy to make and suitable for a Hashimoto's diet. They're naturally sweetened by ripe bananas and contain no refined sugars.

Ingredients:

- 2 ripe bananas, mashed
- 1 cup rolled oats
- 1/4 cup chopped nuts or seeds (walnuts, almonds, or sunflower seeds)
- 1/4 cup raisins or dried cranberries
- 1 teaspoon cinnamon (optional)

Instructions:

1. Preheat the oven to 350°F (175°C) and line a baking sheet with parchment paper.

2. In a mixing bowl, combine mashed bananas, rolled oats, chopped nuts or seeds, raisins or dried cranberries, and cinnamon if using.

3. Drop spoonfuls of the mixture onto the prepared baking sheet, shaping them into cookie rounds.

4. Bake for 12-15 minutes or until the edges are golden brown.

5. Allow the cookies to cool before enjoying.

Cooking Time: 15 minutes

2. Coconut Chia Seed Pudding

This coconut chia seed pudding is a creamy and satisfying dessert option that's rich in fiber and healthy fats. It's naturally sweetened with a touch of maple syrup or honey.

Ingredients:

- 1/4 cup chia seeds
- 1 cup coconut milk (canned or homemade)
- 1 tablespoon maple syrup or honey
- 1/2 teaspoon vanilla extract
- Shredded coconut and fresh berries for topping (optional)

Instructions:

1. In a bowl, mix chia seeds, coconut milk, maple syrup or honey, and vanilla extract. Stir well.

2. Cover and refrigerate the mixture for at least 4 hours or overnight until it thickens into a pudding-like consistency.

3. Before serving, top with shredded coconut and fresh berries if desired.

Cooking Time: 5 minutes (plus refrigeration time)

3. Baked Apples with Cinnamon

These baked apples offer a warm and comforting dessert option without added sugars. The natural sweetness of the apples, enhanced by cinnamon, makes for a delightful treat.

Ingredients:

- Apples (such as Granny Smith or Honeycrisp)
- Cinnamon
- Chopped nuts (optional)

Instructions:

1. Preheat the oven to 375°F (190°C).

2. Core the apples, leaving the bottoms intact to create a well for filling.

3. Sprinkle cinnamon generously over the cored apples and fill the wells with chopped nuts if desired.

4. Place the apples in a baking dish and bake for 20-25 minutes or until tender.

5. Serve the baked apples warm.

Cooking Time: 25 minutes

4. Dark Chocolate Avocado Mousse

This dark chocolate avocado mousse is a creamy and decadent dessert made with nutrient-rich avocados and dark chocolate. It's a guilt-free indulgence suitable for a Hashimoto's diet.

Ingredients:

- 2 ripe avocados
- 1/4 cup unsweetened cocoa powder

- 1/4 cup maple syrup or honey
- 1 teaspoon vanilla extract
- Pinch of salt
- Dark chocolate shavings for garnish (optional)

Instructions:

1. Scoop the flesh of ripe avocados into a blender or food processor.

2. Add cocoa powder, maple syrup or honey, vanilla extract, and a pinch of salt.

3. Blend until smooth and creamy, scraping down the sides as needed.

4. Divide the mousse into serving cups and refrigerate for at least 30 minutes.

5. Garnish with dark chocolate shavings before serving if desired.

Cooking Time: 5 minutes

5. Mixed Berry Frozen Yogurt Bark

This mixed berry frozen yogurt bark is a refreshing and low-sugar dessert option. It's made with Greek yogurt and topped with an assortment of berries for a burst of flavor.

Ingredients:

- 2 cups Greek yogurt (dairy-free if preferred)
- 1 tablespoon honey or maple syrup (optional)
- Mixed berries (blueberries, strawberries, raspberries)
- Shredded coconut or chopped nuts for topping (optional)

Instructions:

1. Line a baking sheet with parchment paper.

2. In a bowl, mix Greek yogurt and honey or maple syrup if using.

3. Spread the yogurt mixture evenly on the parchment paper, about 1/4-inch thick.

4. Sprinkle mixed berries and shredded coconut or chopped nuts on top.

5. Freeze for at least 3 hours or until firm, then break into pieces before serving.

Cooking Time: 3 hours freezing time

These dessert recipes offer delightful and satisfying options while adhering to the principles of a Hashimoto's diet. They incorporate natural sweeteners and nutrient-rich ingredients for a guilt-free and enjoyable dessert experience. Adjust ingredients according to preferences and dietary needs for a delicious treat!

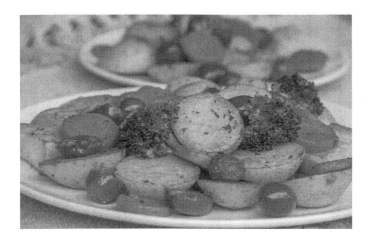

CHAPTER FIVE

Hashimoto Diet Snack Recipes

These snacks focus on providing nutrient-dense options to support thyroid health while being delicious and easy to prepare.

1. Almond Butter Energy Balls

These almond butter energy balls are a convenient and satisfying snack option, rich in protein, healthy fats, and fiber. They're perfect for on-the-go energy and cravings.

Ingredients:

- 1 cup rolled oats
- 1/2 cup almond butter
- 1/4 cup honey or maple syrup
- 1/4 cup shredded coconut (unsweetened)
- 1/4 cup chopped almonds or almond meal
- 1 teaspoon vanilla extract
- Pinch of salt
- Optional add-ins: chia seeds, flaxseeds, or dark chocolate chips

Instructions:

1. In a bowl, mix rolled oats, almond butter, honey or maple syrup, shredded coconut, chopped almonds or almond meal, vanilla extract, and a pinch of salt.

2. If desired, add in any optional add-ins like chia seeds, flaxseeds, or dark chocolate chips.

3. Form the mixture into small balls using your hands.

4. Place the energy balls on a baking sheet lined with parchment paper and refrigerate for at least 30 minutes before enjoying.

Preparation Time: 15 minutes

2. Veggie Sticks with Hummus

This snack pairs colorful vegetable sticks with homemade hummus, providing a satisfying and nutrient-packed option that's rich in vitamins, fiber, and protein.

Ingredients:

- Assorted vegetables (carrots, cucumber, bell peppers)

- 1 can chickpeas, drained and rinsed
- 2 tablespoons tahini
- 2 tablespoons olive oil
- Juice of 1 lemon
- 1 clove garlic, minced
- Salt and pepper to taste

Instructions:

1. Wash and cut assorted vegetables into sticks.

2. In a food processor, blend chickpeas, tahini, olive oil, lemon juice, minced garlic, salt, and pepper until smooth to make the hummus.

3. Serve the vegetable sticks with the homemade hummus for dipping.

Preparation Time: 15 minutes

3. Baked Sweet Potato Chips

These baked sweet potato chips offer a crunchy and healthier alternative to traditional chips. They're rich in vitamins and fiber, making them a perfect snack choice.

Ingredients:

- Sweet potatoes
- Olive oil
- Salt and pepper to taste
- Optional seasoning: paprika, garlic powder, or rosemary

Instructions:

1. Preheat the oven to 375°F (190°C) and line a baking sheet with parchment paper.

2. Wash and peel sweet potatoes, then thinly slice them using a mandoline slicer or knife.

3. Toss the sweet potato slices with olive oil, salt, pepper, and optional seasoning in a bowl until coated.

4. Arrange the slices in a single layer on the prepared baking sheet.

5. Bake for 15-20 minutes, flipping halfway through, until the chips are crispy and lightly browned.

Cooking Time: 20 minutes

4. Greek Yogurt Parfait

This Greek yogurt parfait is a refreshing and protein-rich snack option. It combines the goodness of Greek yogurt with fruits and nuts for a delicious and nutritious treat.

Ingredients:

- Greek yogurt (dairy-free if preferred)
- Mixed berries (blueberries, strawberries, raspberries)
- Chopped nuts (almonds, walnuts)
- Optional: honey or maple syrup for sweetness

Instructions:

1. Layer Greek yogurt, mixed berries, and chopped nuts in a glass or bowl.

2. If desired, drizzle a small amount of honey or maple syrup for added sweetness.

3. Repeat the layers and enjoy this flavorful and satisfying snack.

Preparation Time: 5 minutes

5. Roasted Chickpeas

Roasted chickpeas are a crunchy and flavorful snack loaded with protein and fiber. They're a great alternative to processed snacks, offering a satisfying crunch.

Ingredients:

- 1 can chickpeas, drained and rinsed
- 1 tablespoon olive oil
- Seasonings of choice (such as paprika, cumin, garlic powder)
- Salt and pepper to taste

Instructions:

1. Preheat the oven to 400°F (200°C) and line a baking sheet with parchment paper.

2. Pat dry the chickpeas with a paper towel to remove excess moisture.

3. In a bowl, toss the chickpeas with olive oil, seasonings, salt, and pepper until coated.

4. Spread the chickpeas in a single layer on the prepared baking sheet.

5. Bake for 25-30 minutes, shaking the pan occasionally, until the chickpeas are crispy and golden brown.

Cooking Time: 30 minutes

These snack recipes offer a variety of flavors and nutrients while adhering to the principles of a Hashimoto's diet. They're simple to prepare and can be customized according to preferences and dietary needs for a satisfying snack experience.

Hashimoto Diet Smoothies and Juicing Recipes

1. Green Detox Smoothie

This green detox smoothie is packed with nutrient-dense ingredients that support thyroid health and aid in detoxification.

Ingredients:

- 1 cup spinach
- 1/2 cucumber, chopped
- 1/2 green apple, cored
- 1/2 lemon, juiced
- 1 tablespoon fresh ginger, grated
- 1 cup coconut water or filtered water
- Optional: a handful of fresh mint leaves

Instructions:

1. Place all ingredients in a blender.

2. Blend until smooth and creamy.

3. Pour into a glass and enjoy this refreshing green detox smoothie.

Preparation Time: 5 minutes

2. Berry Blast Smoothie

This berry blast smoothie is rich in antioxidants and vitamins, making it a delicious and nutritious choice for a Hashimoto's diet.

Ingredients:

- 1 cup mixed berries (strawberries, blueberries, raspberries)
- 1/2 banana
- 1/2 cup Greek yogurt (dairy-free if preferred)
- 1 tablespoon chia seeds
- 1 cup almond milk or any preferred milk

Instructions:

1. Combine all ingredients in a blender.

2. Blend until smooth and well-combined.

3. Pour into a glass and savor this flavorful berry blast smoothie.

Preparation Time: 5 minutes

3. Pineapple Turmeric Anti-Inflammatory Juice

This pineapple turmeric juice is a powerful anti-inflammatory drink that can aid in reducing inflammation associated with Hashimoto's disease.

Ingredients:

- 2 cups fresh pineapple chunks
- 1-inch piece of fresh turmeric root (or 1 teaspoon ground turmeric)
- 1-inch piece of fresh ginger
- 1 lemon, juiced
- Pinch of black pepper (helps with turmeric absorption)
- 1-2 cups filtered water or coconut water

Instructions:

1. Juice the pineapple, turmeric root, ginger, and lemon using a juicer.

2. Transfer the juice to a blender, add a pinch of black pepper, and blend briefly.

3. Strain the juice through a fine-mesh sieve to remove any pulp.

4. Dilute with filtered water or coconut water to reach the desired consistency.

5. Serve this anti-inflammatory juice immediately over ice.

Preparation Time: 10 minutes

4. Tropical Mango Banana Smoothie

This tropical mango banana smoothie is a delightful and creamy drink loaded with vitamins and minerals, perfect for a Hashimoto's diet.

Ingredients:

- 1 ripe mango, peeled and chopped
- 1 ripe banana
- 1/2 cup coconut milk or almond milk
- 1/4 cup Greek yogurt (dairy-free if preferred)
- 1 tablespoon honey or maple syrup (optional)
- Ice cubes (if desired)

Instructions:

1. Combine all ingredients in a blender.

2. Blend until smooth and creamy.

3. Add ice cubes if a colder consistency is desired.

4. Pour into a glass and enjoy this tropical mango banana smoothie.

Preparation Time: 5 minutes

5. Beetroot Carrot Ginger Juice

This beetroot carrot ginger juice is a vibrant and nutrient-packed drink that's beneficial for boosting immunity and supporting thyroid health.

Ingredients:

- 2 medium-sized beetroots, peeled and chopped
- 3 medium-sized carrots, washed and chopped
- 1-inch piece of fresh ginger
- 1 apple, cored
- 1 lemon, juiced
- 1-2 cups filtered water or coconut water

Instructions:

1. Juice the beetroots, carrots, ginger, apple, and lemon using a juicer.

2. Strain the juice through a fine-mesh sieve to remove any pulp.

3. Dilute with filtered water or coconut water as desired.

4. Serve this vibrant beetroot carrot ginger juice immediately.

Preparation Time: 10 minutes

These smoothies and juice recipes offer a range of flavors and nutrients, aligning with the principles of a Hashimoto's diet. They're simple to prepare and can be customized according to personal preferences for a refreshing and healthful experience.

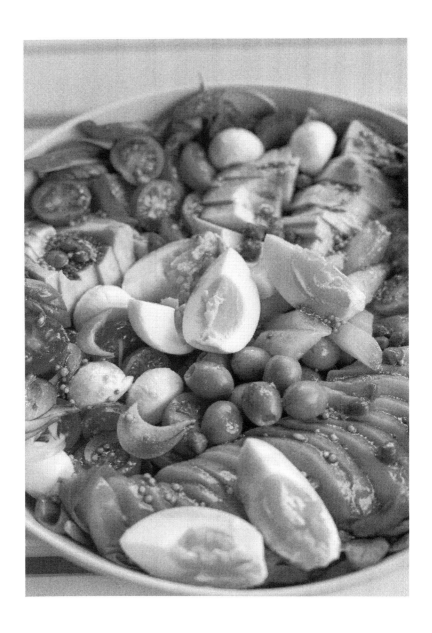

CONCLUSION

Crafting a tailored diet to support individuals with Hashimoto's disease requires a thoughtful blend of nutritious, flavorful, and thyroid-friendly recipes. Throughout this culinary journey, a careful selection of ingredients, mindful cooking methods, and a focus on nutrient-rich foods have been the guiding principles.

Embracing a Hashimoto disease diet isn't solely about restriction but rather about nourishing the body with foods that foster well-being, mitigate symptoms, and support overall thyroid health.

These recipes represent a harmonious fusion of taste and health, ensuring that every meal or snack is a step towards optimal wellness. The Hashimoto's diet isn't a rigid prescription but rather a flexible approach to accommodate individual needs while aligning with the foundational principles of the condition.

In exploring breakfast options, the recipes prioritized a balance of protein, healthy fats, and complex carbohydrates. From chia seed puddings to savory omelets, each morning meal aimed to kickstart the day with energy and sustenance while incorporating ingredients beneficial for thyroid function.

Lunchtime offered a spectrum of dishes, from quinoa salads to hearty soups. These meals were designed to be wholesome, providing essential nutrients to maintain energy levels throughout the day. By focusing on lean proteins, vegetables, and healthy grains, these lunches catered to a balanced diet that contributes positively to thyroid health.

Dinner recipes aimed to conclude the day with satiating yet nutritious meals. Baked salmon, stuffed bell peppers, and vegetable curries brought an array of flavors while incorporating ingredients rich in essential vitamins and minerals. These dinners were crafted not just to fill the stomach but to support the body's nutritional requirements, promoting well-being and aiding in managing Hashimoto's disease.

The dessert options presented a delightful balance between health-conscious choices and satisfying cravings. By embracing natural sweeteners and wholesome ingredients, the dessert recipes allowed individuals to indulge in guilt-free treats, whether it was through baked apples, chia seed puddings, or dark chocolate avocado mousse.

Snack options aimed to bridge the gap between meals with nourishing bites that maintained energy levels and supported the body's nutritional demands. From almond butter energy balls to roasted chickpeas, these snacks were designed to be convenient, satisfying, and aligned with the principles of a Hashimoto's diet.

Furthermore, the inclusion of smoothies and juicing recipes expanded the horizons of nutrient intake. These vibrant concoctions of fruits, vegetables, and superfoods were aimed at boosting immunity, reducing inflammation, and providing a refreshing and convenient way to consume vital nutrients.

In essence, the Hashimoto's disease diet recipes offered an array of options to transform eating habits into a proactive approach toward wellness. Beyond just recipes, they symbolize a commitment to nourishing the body, supporting thyroid health, and embracing a lifestyle that fosters vitality and balance.

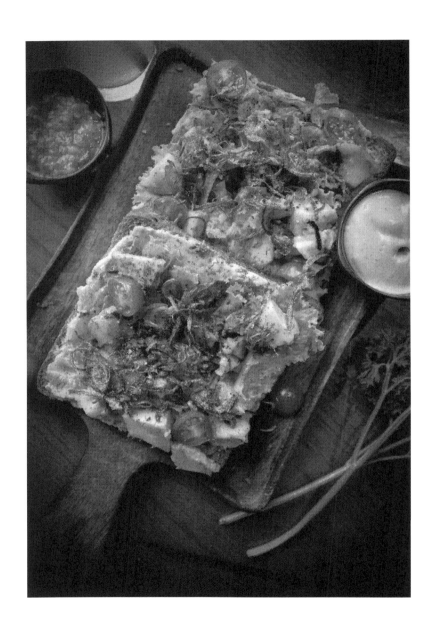

Printed by Amazon Italia Logistica S.r.l.
Torrazza Piemonte (TO), Italy

56270972R00042